Diet and Nutrition

A Dietary Guide
By Martin J. Hibbs

First published 2014
This edition
Produced by
Martin J. Hibbs
© 2018

Disclaimer

Please note - Whilst the author of this guide is a qualified dietician, he is not a qualified medical practitioner or physician; therefore where any medical conditions are referred to and nutritional advice given, this is done on the understanding that the reader of this document will keep their general medical practitioner informed in respect to any illnesses they might suffer and will consult with them in respect to a suitable treatment rather than simply rely upon the information given in this publication.

It is also important to note that any guidance given in this book is general in nature and freely available from many sources, therefore such guidance should not be directly attributed to the author.

This guide is not a definitive guide to diet and nutrition. Whilst every effort has been made to keep this book up to date and as accurate as possible; dietary advice tends to change frequently over time. Because of this fact; neither the author, publishers, nor the distributors of this book can accept any liability in respect to any information deemed to be misleading or inaccurate in this publication.

After reading this book, and in order to find out more about diet and nutrition, or a specific health issue mentioned in this publication, it is advisable to cross reference any information given with other books of a similar nature. Where health matters are concerned, it is always important to get the very latest, most accurate, and up to date information on any given health condition possible (preferably, directly from a doctor or professionally recognised healthcare professional).

DIET AND NUTRITION

INDEX

	Page No
INTRODUCTION.	9
AUTHOR'S GUIDANCE NOTES.	11 - 23
DEFINITION OF NUTRITION	23 - 25
A BALANCED DIET	25 - 39
General health diet	38 - 41
NUTRITION IN RESPECT TO LIFESTAGES	43 – 50
Pregnancy	50 - 58
Babies/Children	58 - 62
Teenagers / Clerical Workers	62 - 66
Manual Labourers/Sports Persons	66 - 71
Female complications - Old Age	71 - 74

DIET AND NUTRITION

INDEX

	Page No
SPECIALISED DIETS	74 - 87
Digestive Disorders	87 - 90
Dairy-Free Diet Options	90 - 91
Low Calorie Options	91 - 96
PERSONAL CIRCUMSTANCES.	92 - 106
ORGANIC OR MASS PRODUCED	106 - 110
PROBLEM FOODS	110 - 118
BUYER BEWARE.	118 - 124
MINERAL / VITAMIN INDEX	124 - 129
VEGETARIAN DIETS	105 - 109
SLIMMING AND EXERCISE.	129 – 40
CLOSING STATEMENT	141

INTRODUCTION

In today's hectic world, few of us give any thought to the long-term implications of our diets and yet the food we eat (like the fuel we put into our vehicles) will determine our bodily performance for the rest of our lives.

Whilst we may not be consciously aware of it, the way we think, our actions and bodily efficiency are all determined by the foods we put into our mouths. In some cases we consume stimulants such as coffee for example, which like other stimulants, can send our minds and bodies racing. In some cases, such stimulants can contribute to negative emotional states such as anger hyperactivity etc.

In other cases foods can make us lethargic (particularly fats when consumed to excess); certain types of food can be acidic too, which may cause or aggravate conditions such as arthritis. Failure to eat the right kinds of food can therefore have the most serious of implications for us all, bringing about illness, even death in some cases (as a result of heart disease, strokes etc).

Our bodies are a very complex blend of cellular, chemical and mechanical interactions, all of which need specific types of fuel to interact successfully. It is also a fact that our nutritional needs change and vary greatly, according to our life-stages and lifestyles. It is therefore essential that we know a little about (and understand) the role and effects which certain foodstuffs play in our lives if we are all to remain healthy.

All too often we eat to satisfy ourselves emotionally, rather than to nourish ourselves physically. In a good many cases we have little or no knowledge in respect to the foodstuffs we consume, or their effects upon our bodies.

The aim of this guide is to give sufficient information so that you the reader can make informed choices in respect to your diet, and where necessary, make any required adjustments using the guidelines contained in this document.

AUTHOR'S GUIDANCE NOTES

As the title suggests, this dietary guide has been written to assist those who wish to maintain a healthy lifestyle. It covers most areas and caters for most dietary needs and requirements in respect to each life-stage and lifestyle. It should however be noted that this guide covers the principle of diet and nutrition in basic terms only.

Where diet plans are suggested, please note these are intended merely as helpful suggestions only. Before embarking on any specific diet, you should always consult your regular medical practitioner (someone who knows your medical history in great detail and can spot any potential flaws in your proposed dietary path) or a qualified dietician.

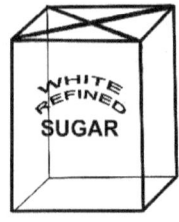 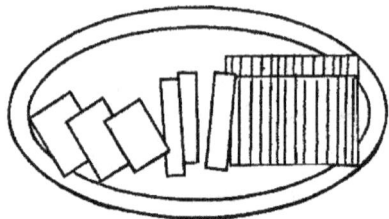

    Those wishing to know more in respect to specific areas of diet and nutrition as outlined in this guide, i.e. calorie assessment/management, the chemical components of foodstuffs etc would be well advised to approach their local dietician/health centre. Alternatively, you also have the option of visiting local bookstores, where some very good guides can be found these days, guides which cover such issues in greater depth. Another alternative can be to use the internet for research purposes, you can then print off any useful information you find.

    The diet plan examples included in this document are designed not so much with calorific value in mind, but more for nutritional content. This is why items such as coffee, white sugar, white bread, sweets and cakes are not included in any of the following plans, as it is known their nutritional value is very low. Where such foods are consumed, they should only be eaten in very small quantities. Even as part of an apparently healthy person's diet, they could potentially cause some kind of ill health if consumed in large amounts.

Please note also* where possible meal plans in this document are concerned; these are based upon the assumption that those using them are in good health, with no food intolerance problems; i.e. in respect to wheat, milk based foods, nut allergies etc. Also in respect to the meal-plans contained in this document; it is essential that the meal examples given are varied and NOT JUST ONE OF THE FOODS/ITEMS ON THE LIST chosen time after time and eaten repeatedly (see problem foods further on in this document).

If when reading the diet ideas in this book, you acknowledge a health problem, such as diabetes, heart problems, or in respect to cereal or lactose intolerance etc, then some of the examples given in the following plans may not be suitable for you.

In this case another more tailored diet-plan will be needed, one specifically made for such conditions. Where high sugar or cholesterol foods are concerned; some of the options given in the general health diet plan would most definitely not be suitable in such cases.

The foods in the plans are also intended to be readily available at supermarkets, meaning that their exact makeup can vary, i.e. the quality of the ingredients can vary, in respect to food quality **(see problem foods and Organic or Mass Produced pages)**.

When constructing this guide, it was my original intention that the diet-plans included in later pages would apply in respect to home prepared foods, where quality could be overseen, but sadly with modern busy lifestyles, home-cooking is far less commonplace. This being the case, supermarkets and mass food producers have now stepped in to fill this need in respect to pies, puddings, cooked meats, and other major meal components.

Where some foods in the diet plans occur, i.e. chips, chocolate bars, bacon, ham, pies with pastry etc, a degree of caution and common sense needs to be applied. Such foods certainly fit in the problem foods category, but in small amounts they can be consumed under the "**a little bit** of what you fancy does you good" principle. That said however, **such foods should most definitely be eaten in moderation and in small portions with other good foods,** i.e. with salads etc.

All the foods mentioned in the following plans are recommended to maintain optimum health in respect to each life stage or situation. Strict calorie plans have purposely been omitted from this document in the knowledge that few people can stick to them.

To some, this may seem like a defeatist attitude, but the reality of the issue is this: To be successful, a diet must be palatable so that the person undertaking it does not get bored with it, or become disheartened as a result of severe restrictions put upon them.

When someone undertakes a controlled diet, there is generally a sound reason for doing so. We are all human and likely to transgress on occasion, and so to set difficult or unrealistic calorie based targets could easily undermine a person's chances of achieving their goal. If our confidence is so undermined by unrealistic targets that we abandon our diet, then the threat to our health will be that much greater (especially if a diet is on medical grounds).

The odd transgression can be catered for. Whilst this might mean being on a restricted dietary regime for longer, this is far more preferable than having to abandon the project altogether, simply because of slight deviations, i.e. the odd chocolate bar or cake. Sadly deviations are likely to occur on occasion.

Items such as chocolate, cakes etc, may possibly be too tempting to resist, or be a necessary pick me up from time to time; this being the case, allowances have been made for such deviations when drawing up each of the following plans. This does not give the person on a diet the licence to eat as they please however, but merely is meant as a form of reassurance to aid a person in their goal. Ultimately it is far better to resist temptation of course, as required results will show themselves that much quicker.

In order to keep dietary deviations to a minimum, it is important to vary the choice and cooking style of the foods mentioned in the following plans. This should help in respect to observance of any recommended diet plan we choose to undertake.

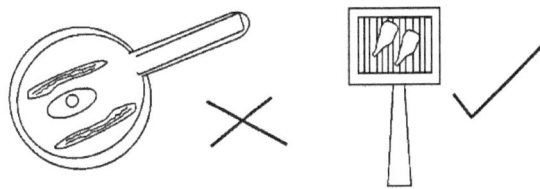

As regards cooking styles; the frying of foods is not recommended when one wishes to lose weight. Ideally, meat etc should be grilled (so as to remove as much fat as possible).

In the few cases where chips etc are fried, it is best to leave them to drain by placing them on a piece of kitchen roll, which will absorb any excess fat or oil from the cooking process employed. As regards vegetables - they should be boiled on a low heat for as short a time as possible, that way they will retain most of their goodness.

As regards the calorific values for each diet plan mentioned in this book; exact figures for each meal have been purposely omitted, since such details are variable, and need to be amended depending upon how the food is prepared, e.g. fried, poached, grilled etc. It is also the case that average portions can vary greatly from person to person.

In the case of those who wish to stick to a calorie plan of some kind, it is worth noting that most food manufacturers give clear details as regards to the nutrients and calorific values in respect to their products on the packaging of their products. Sadly we cannot easily live on these products alone however; where possible, meats, vegetables and dairy products should all be a part of a persons' diet if they are to stay healthy (see vegetarian section) unless a certain foodstuff causes known health issues. As I've stated above, the calorie and nutrient value of these foods very much depends upon how they are prepared.

Another common area where problems can arise with calorific values, lies in respect to knowing those foods which have the highest amount of calories.

As a task, calorie assessment can certainly be a very difficult one in that logical assessment does not always work (the most surprising of foods can be high in calories). Published calorie guides listing the calorific values of foods can therefore prove invaluable when calorie counting is an issue of great importance.

Fortunately calorie guides are readily available in most bookshops, health/health-food shops via the internet etc, and are often very reasonably priced, depending upon their quality (or for free if you use the internet).

Thanks to medical science, we now have far greater knowledge as regards our various life-stages and circumstances and so we are in a better position to look after ourselves. We are after all what we eat. If we eat properly, according to our individual `contracting many of the illnesses which have cut the lives of others tragically short in the past, i.e. heart attacks and strokes etc.

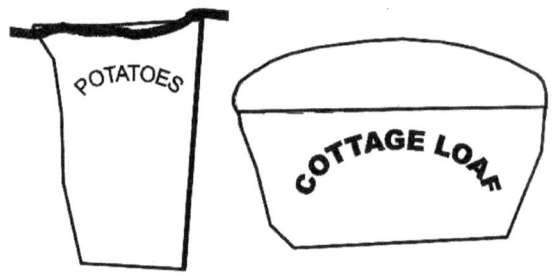

    The bulk of a person's diet should ideally come in carbohydrate form i.e. pasta, bread, rice potatoes or plain biscuits. Although these foodstuffs are moderately low in saturated fats they are still a good source of energy.

    Where bread is concerned, it is best to go for brown wholemeal varieties, since the white options have often been bleached and lost most of their goodness during production. In the case of white bread, much of the necessary fibre has also been lost, leaving it in a stodgy form, which is known to be very bad for the digestive system. When sandwiches etc are mentioned in this dietary guide they should therefore be made from the more natural (less refined) options that are available. Alternatively as a compromise, by way of 50/50 bread that is now widely available and which does at least offer some benefit in respect to fibre content.

Whether we are planning our own diet or planning someone else's, it is necessary to take account of lifestyle as well as life-stage and where possible, guard against likely health problems.

In the main, people suffering from nutritional deficiencies **feel run down, i.e. they look pale and generally feel very weak, or tired.** Should these symptoms occur, a visit to a healthcare professional is often a good idea. Where necessary they will arrange for a simple blood test to be carried out, once the results are known, any nutrient deficiencies can be quickly addressed.

Many illnesses are the result of a poor diet over many years, i.e. arthritis, tooth decay, hair frailty and poor eyesight etc; though genetic disposition can also play a part of course. It is therefore important to take these common illnesses into account when planning our diets; tooth decay is a perfect example of providing for each life-stage.

Our teeth will only stand so many

refined, high sugared, foodstuffs. It's true we can replace our teeth artificially, however such replacements never compare with those with which we are born. Likewise with eyesight, in respect to optical glasses - prevention of illness is therefore far better than a repaired or modified organ.

It should also be noted that where salads are recommended in this document, salad dressings should be avoided or used to a minimum, as they are known to be high in calories (even some low calorie versions, can have an unreasonable amount of calories in some cases).

Where the dairy free diet options are given on later pages, it should be noted that these options are merely basic examples. There are a great many official vegetarian foods/meals to choose from as well. There are also many informative vegetarian cookbooks/dietary books available for reference at our local bookshops/libraries and online too.

THE DEFINITION OF NUTRITION

Before going on to describe the nutritional needs of each life-stage, it is first important to understand the word nutrition, and also to define a balanced diet.

Nutrition: The definition of this word, being food for promoting growth and repair of living tissues - whether in reference to a single plant cell or a complex group of cells such as mankind - in order to sustain life.

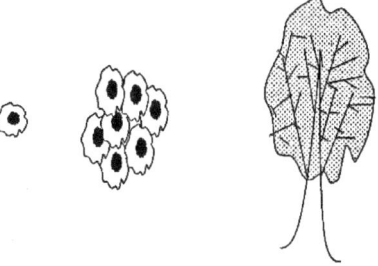

The nutrients required to sustain life can vary tremendously in substance. The most common requirements are oxygen, nitrogen and water, though it can be said that in some species, carbon dioxide (a human waste product), heat and light are also essential, since they act as catalysts with other nutrient components.

Many nutritional components are obtained directly from the soil (which sustains most life forces in one way or another). For example, most of the minerals and trace elements we humans depend on, come from plant structures which we hopefully consume on a regular basis, i.e. cabbage, beans, peas, lettuce and root vegetables, which use the said minerals and trace elements to sustain their own life force.

Nutrients generally enter the body orally and voluntarily, though in certain cases, i.e. illness or through accidental damage, food is placed strategically around the body via drips and medicine, to be broken down and used immediately. This indicates that food is not necessarily of a solid state, and quantity of meal does not necessarily relate to performance and nourishment.

The latter example of nutritional supply in extreme circumstances leads me on to the next matter of defining a balanced diet.

A BALANCED DIET

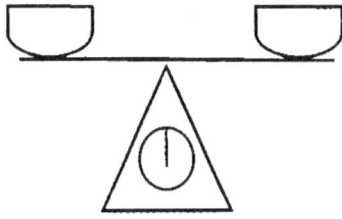

A balanced diet is a series of small meals, designed to give adequate nutritional value from a range of foodstuffs (that will hopefully be palatable to the recipient). A balanced diet allows us to keep our body tissue in as near perfect health as is possible, whilst at the same time providing us with sufficient energy fuel so that we can undertake our normal duties in life.

Under normal circumstances a meal should contain an equal amount of proteins, fats and carbohydrates, though as I will explain later, this criteria varies according to a person's way of life and life-stage position. Of these three vital components, proteins are by far the most important since they make up the body tissue itself; they are in effect the body's building blocks and should be an essential part of any meal.

Although the body has the ability to convert any excess protein into fuel (by way of storing it as body fat reserves), it is unable to manufacture protein itself from either of the other main components (i.e. fats and carbohydrates). Our protein reserves therefore depend upon our consumption of them on a regular basis. Fortunately for us, proteins are easily obtained, the most common source being animal derivatives, i.e. meat, eggs, fish, dairy produce, seafood; and vegetable sources, i.e. cereals, nuts and beans.

Each of these foodstuffs contribute their own particular type of protein (of which there are many). That is why they should all be consumed on a regular basis (unless otherwise directed by our physician), since they are in effect the central pivot of our dietary needs. Although these foodstuffs can be bad for us if eaten to excess, they are all necessary in their own way to replace the various proteins which are being used up in the never-ending process of growth and repair to our bodies which takes place.

Whilst it's true that excess protein is likely to be laid down as fat, too little will most certainly upset the balance of one's diet irreparably and bring about serious physical dysfunction within our bodies.

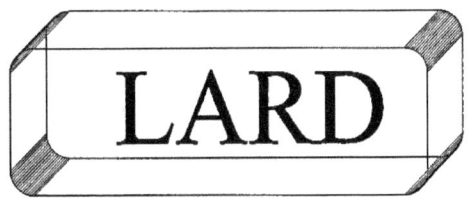

Fats are likewise a very important part of a person's diet and can be classified in two ways, saturated fats and unsaturated fats. Saturated fats are much thicker, hence their tendency to solidify. They are found largely in animal-derived foods (dairy produce etc). Whilst we need a small proportion of these fats for insulation, they are on the whole bad for us and care should be taken to restrict the amount we have in each meal. Over-consumption of such material can lead to diseases such as atherosclerosis (congestion of the main artery, caused by fatty deposits), leading to hear attacks and strokes. Over-consumption is also heavily implicated in certain types of cancer too.

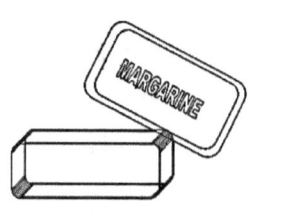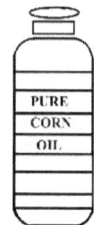

Unsaturated fats are a different matter altogether. They are an essential ingredient of each meal, since they provide us with fuel. They are also very important in respect to the metabolism of the brain and nervous system.

When calculating a diet plan it must be remembered that we burn up many calories via the autonomic nervous system (i.e. digestive organs, cardiac and reproductive organs), none of these we consciously think of as being highly expendable of energy.

Even in our sleep, life and subconscious bodily functions are still going on as normal if you think about it; we must therefore take these systems into consideration when structuring our diets.

Besides providing essential fuel, unsaturated fats help to displace and transport saturated fats around the body, thus helping to prevent the clogging up of our arteries (round the heart for example). Unsaturated fats, as previously stated, are found mainly in vegetable oils and in fish, (also to some degree in nuts and pulses), remaining in a liquefied state even at low temperature.

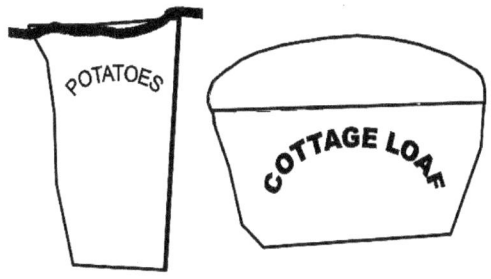

The third major dietary ingredient we need to include in our diet are carbohydrates, which provide the bulk of our energy needs, both thermal (heat producing), and kinetic (movement energy). Carbohydrates occur in our diet either as a form of sugar, i.e. glucose (the major fuel the body uses), or as starch, i.e. potatoes, pasta and bread, which although requiring more complex processing, still provide us with large amounts of energy.

As well as sugar and starch there is a third member of the carbohydrate group which is cellulose, a material which we cannot actually digest, but which does form a valuable part of our diet in that it helps and improves peristalsis (digestion). Cellulose occurs mainly in cereal, bran and the leaves of certain vegetables, i.e. lettuce and cabbage. Carbohydrates are without doubt the cheapest source of energy and form the basis of most diets.

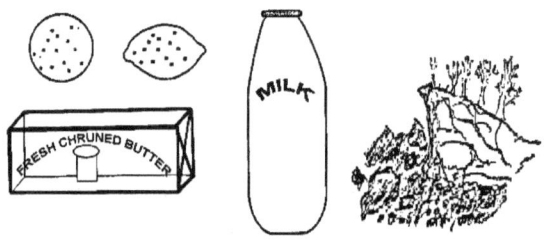

As well as proteins, fats and carbohydrates it should be noted that vitamins, minerals and trace elements should also be taken into account when constructing a balanced diet.

Vitamins need to be understood and monitored in each meal, since they have great influence upon the body via the glandular system.

Most people know of **vitamin C** and its importance to the lymphatic system and have read of deficiency diseases such as scurvy. Similarly, most people are familiar with **vitamin D** which is necessary for strong bones and teeth (a deficiency will lead to brittle bones or rickets).

The need for **vitamin A (retinol)** found in carrots, has also been much publicised for maintaining good eyesight and night vision. What is not so well known is that **vitamin A**, plays a major role in the health of our external body tissue, i.e. our hair, skin and nails etc. These three vitamins however, account for only a small proportion of our vitamin requirements.

There is, for example the vitamin B group, comprising of at least 9 vitamins. They play a major part in carbohydrate metabolism, and the blood composition of our bodies. They also help to regulate the nervous system.

The major vitamins in this group are **B1 (thiamine), B2 (riboflavin), B5, B6, B12, folic acid, pantothenic acid, niacin, biotin, and choline,** which deals with fat metabolism. The other main vitamins are **K** and **E**, which also regulate blood metabolism.

These vitamins are to be found in many different sources, i.e. **vitamin A** can be found in green vegetables, fruit, fish oils, and dairy produce. The **vitamin B group** are found mostly in meat and cereals. **Vitamin C** as we know is found mainly in fresh fruit and vegetables, as are folic acids (mainly in oranges, blackcurrants and green vegetables). **Vitamin D** is to be found in butter, margarine, animal and vegetable oils and fresh fish. **Vitamin E** is to be found in bread and cereals, fresh vegetables and also fruit. **Vitamin K** is found mainly in leafy vegetables.

Traditionally, dieticians have recommended that we try to eat five portions of fresh fruit and vegetables a day, with some now recommending that we have seven per day. Whilst five portions can seem a lot, seven may seem unreasonable to many. Most importantly, what we have to take into account however is the type of fruit and vegetables we chose to eat.

It is for example perfectly acceptable

to have a plate of mixed vegetables (cost allowing) rather than say a plate of just peas. It is also very important to realise that our choice of fruit is very important too. If for example we try to eat too many citrus type fruits, i.e. oranges, grapefruits or strawberries, or these types of fruit juices, this can have an adverse affect upon us.

Being acid based fruits, if taken in too large a dose, they can cause us digestive illnesses such as stomach ulcers, indigestion or Irritable Bowel Syndrome.

It is however fairly straightforward for us to buy a pack of mixed fruit (preferably unsweetened) and stick to eating apples, pears, bananas and maybe eat a few dried apricots or dates as a snack. Not only are dates and apricots very nutritious, they are also very high in fibre. (This option is not advisable for diabetics however.)

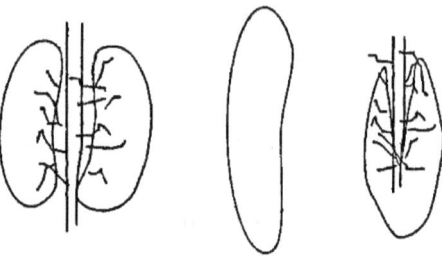

One very efficient way to be sure we get essential vitamins can be to include liver or kidneys in our diet plan, since most animal liver and kidneys contain very large amounts of the said vitamins. (This option does not suite everyone's taste though.)

The final components of a balanced diet not yet covered are minerals and trace elements.

Minerals and trace elements are usually soil derived. They become part of our diet via soil grown crops, i.e. greens and fruit. We are also able to get these elements via animal produce and fish, from creatures which during their lives have eaten green matter that is soil or silt derived, in order to maintain their own body tissue.

These minerals are also the basis of our own bodies of course - **magnesium;**

calcium and phosphorus for example are the main constituents of our skeletal system. We also use these minerals in our soft tissue, along with **chlorine, sodium** and **potassium**, which regulate and control our cell structure, i.e. temperature control and nutrient absorption.

Magnesium and **Sulphur** play an important part in the brain and nervous system, both in electrical conductivity **(magnesium)** and in protecting the nerve tissue from infection **(sulphur)**. **Iron**, as is well known, is the major constituent of haemoglobin in the blood and is found in meat products. Besides these major minerals, there are also trace elements to take into account. Whilst they are only required in very small amounts, they still play their part.

Iodine is very important indeed, since it is an essential part of hormones, produced by the thyroid gland in the neck (these are largely responsible for our metabolism).

Other trace elements are **zinc** (an important accessory to the lymphatic system), **chromium** (which helps us utilise glucose), and **selenium** which helps enzymes in our red blood cells. **Manganese** and **copper** are both associated with enzymes in the body. **It is important to note, however, that absorbing these minerals in too high a dose can prove detrimental to our health, and in extreme cases could prove fatal.**

The final equation in a balanced diet is that of calorific values (i.e. units of energy which the body requires for our ideal metabolic function, both mental and physical). As I have already outlined, they are generally attained both from carbohydrate sources and also fats (of which there are two types, i.e. saturates and unsaturates).

Whilst we do indeed need these valuable constituents in our diet, if taken to excess they are counterproductive and can be responsible for many serious diseases. Therefore we must monitor and regulate their intake, so as to avoid their damaging our health.

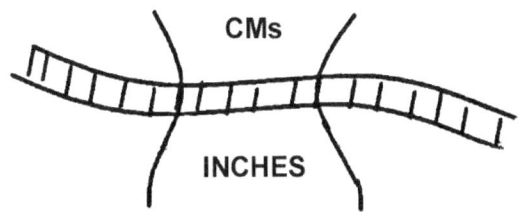

In recent times we have developed a precise measuring procedure for each foodstuff and the units of energy it produces. We have therefore been able to establish (through scientific means) our exact metabolic needs for each life-stage and style as regards these units.

We have learned for example, how unrefined dairy produce, saturated fats and sugars have exceptionally high amounts of energy potential, which, in view of our more sedentary lifestyle these days, we are unlikely to realise. If taken to excess, they are likely to pose a serious health problem to certain categories of the population **(see also problem foods)**. That is not to say we must avoid them, but that we must be wary of them, in terms of the amount we consume.

GENERAL DIET

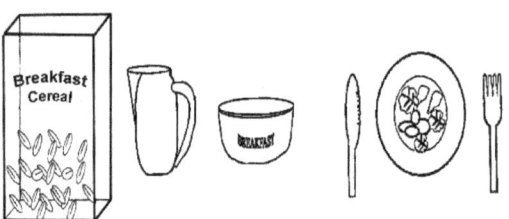

Those with health problems should beware of the meat and dairy options listed below, also those with food intolerances and digestive issues should avoid certain acid foods and fruit juices of the type mentioned below. Please choose suitable alternatives instead.

SUGGESTED BEVERAGES:

Fruit juice, e.g. apple, orange, blackcurrant, milk, mineral water, tea (preferably herb, i.e. mint, rosehip, camomile or green tea).

SUGGESTED BREAKFAST:

Cereal flakes, (preferably unsweetened) compressed wheat bars, or bran, mixed cereals, i.e. muesli.

Crispbread with tomato.

Boiled egg. or fruit.

Thinly buttered toast (with or without egg).

SUGGESTED LUNCH:

Bread roll with various fillings e.g. salad, cheese, ham **(with excess fat removed)** or chicken, **(preferably without skin).**

Baked potatoes with filling (as for roll).

Soup. or beans on toast.

SUGGESTED EVENING MEAL OPTIONS:

Macaroni cheese, boiled potatoes, greens, meat, e.g. liver, kidneys (lamb), shepherds pie.

Salad (with pasta, nuts, chicken or fish).

Sardines on toast.

Steak and kidney pie, with potatoes and vegetables.

Spaghetti bolognaise **(preferably home made with good quality ingredients bought from local suppliers wherever possible)**.

SUGGESTED SWEETS: (if required) - fresh fruit, cooked fruit pie, milk pudding, yoghurt.

NUTRITION IN RESPECT TO LIFE-STAGES

Our nutritional requirements can and do vary greatly depending upon our circumstances. It is also a fact that we require different types of foodstuffs, according to our life-stages (from pregnancy/childhood right through to old age). As well as covering the various life-stages, the following pages will show how our health and performance can be affected, or if necessary, improved.

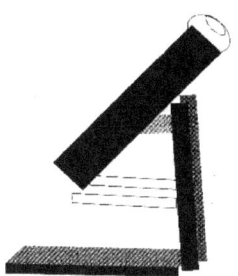

Fortunately for us, our nutritional needs have been the subject of much study and research over the years. As well as having the literature assembled by our forefathers to guide us, we now have the benefit of modern technology to help us work out our exact dietary requirements too. It has been found for example that the average man requires around 2000 -2500 calories per day, whilst the average woman requires around 1800-2000. This does very much depend upon a person's age, lifestyle, working circumstances and personal metabolism however. We all process food differently.

As I mentioned earlier, we now have some very precise measuring devices at our disposal, which can help us to measure the exact intake of certain nutritional materials, and also, the amount of nutritional imbalance within our bodies. We have learned from our forefathers that we must plan for each stage of our life - from conception, right through to the end of our lives.

Nutrition for Pregnancy

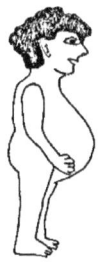

Assuming a pregnancy is planned it is advisable for both partners to eat sensibly prior to conception, with the prospective mother attending a suitable medical clinic. to assess her own health, and any imbalance in her vitamin and mineral levels, i.e. iron, or B complex vitamins. It is wise to adjust both partner's diets where needed, well in advance of conception to avoid the stress of withdrawal symptoms once the mother has conceived, e.g. caffeine and alcohol.

By the time conception has occurred, most bad dietary habits will hopefully have been dealt with (including smoking if applicable).

Pregnancy is a time when it is particularly important to eat a well balanced diet for the mother's sake and that of the developing foetus. There is no need to eat for two however since the baby draws all it needs from the mother's more than adequate nutrient reserves, and excesses of diet by the mother will still result in unhealthy weight gain (putting stress on her heart etc). Despite her current situation, it is of course essential that the mother-to-be observes standard diet procedure regarding her pregnancy, as certain nutrients are essential for the growth and development of a healthy baby and should be included in her daily diet.

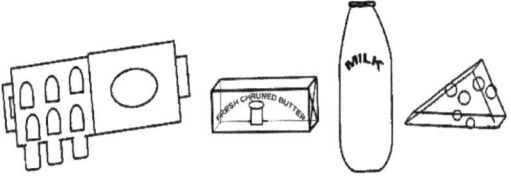

A wide selection of proteins are very important at this stage, both for the growth and development of the baby, and for combating the considerable strain and wear on the mother's own body at this time. Similarly a reasonable intake of iron will be required, since the baby's requirement for iron will be very high and crucial for the formation of red blood cells (for both mother and child).

An iron deficiency at this time could be very serious, since it is the blood which carries all the major nutrients round both bodies and also the waste products to the excretory organs.

Calcium like iron, is also an essential mineral at such times, being necessary to develop the baby's skeletal system. Both will be taken from the mother's reserves and so she needs to ensure that she eats ample amounts of dairy products, provided she has no intolerance issues. As well as being high in calcium, these also provide many of the other minerals, trace elements and vitamins, which will be required

Although a prospective mother may normally be weight conscious, she must realise that dairy products are essential for the wellbeing and development of the baby. If however the expectant mother has been advised by her chosen medical practitioner to avoid such foods on medical grounds, or because she has a strong dislike to such foods, then she can obtain ample calcium from other sources such as tinned sardines, fruit and fresh vegetables. In addition to calcium, vitamin D will also be required. Vitamin D can be found in dairy produce (also in margarine if dairy produce is unsuitable due to lactose intolerance).

During pregnancy it is very important to drink an adequate amount of fluids (preferably mineral water) as this will help to flush any potentially harmful toxins out of the mother's body. As well as helping the foetus, this will also help the mother to stay healthier, since her lymphatic system will be less tied up in dealing with toxins and more able to deal with any infections or viruses she encounters.

Whilst there are no hard and fast dietary rules for pregnancy, if a moderately high dairy diet is chosen, it would be wise to monitor the intake of saturated fats and refined foods (e.g. sugary or high fat) so as to ensure that harmful dietary excess will not occur, either in respect to yourself, or the developing baby. This particularly applies in respect to pregnancy cravings where a hypnotic preference for one, or a series of particular foodstuffs, often occurs. Such cravings often involve one of these two types of high calorific foodstuffs in one form or another (i.e. chocolate etcetera).

In the case of pregnancy, it should also be taken into account that a percentage of pregnant women encounter morning sickness in the early stages of their pregnancy. This has been considered when drawing up the general health diet plan on later pages, which is made up from a selection of foods designed to be palatable should such symptoms occur.

These foods would be suitable, both during, and after pregnancy, though it would be wise to increase the iron content by eating more lean meat and fresh vegetables where possible (vegetarian mums to be, may be able to get sufficient B group vitamins, Iron etc from fresh vegetable and nut sources alone, but careful supervision by a medical practitioner would be a wise precaution in this situation).

During pregnancy it is also advisable to avoid main animal organs such as liver, kidneys etc, since they contain very concentrated forms of vitamins and minerals, which could in some cases, upset the nutrient balance within our own body. (This can also apply in the case of unsupervised supplement intake of course.)

With all the scares that have occurred in recent times, it is only right to give a few words of warning regarding certain foodstuffs and pregnancy. Naturally when pregnant, it is very dangerous for the baby to ignore such things as sell-by dates and cooking instructions (e.g. pre-cooked foods, pork and poultry particularly).

It is also unwise to eat types of pate, raw/not fully cooked eggs/food products, also certain cheeses such as Brie and Camembert, and natural untreated yoghurts, since these have on rare occasions been linked with food poisoning scares.

It is also very important to be wary in the case of pre-packed chilled salad products too (either in mixed or singular form), since they are also of a processed type where bacteria can enter the food chain (i.e. listeria). Where they are purchased, it is essential that they are washed and thoroughly rinsed before they are eaten.

When on holiday overseas, it is also very important to beware of disease potential in respect to salad and water hygiene, as some very harmful diseases can be found overseas. Where others prepare such foods for us, they may be used to such bugs and not so wary of them.

     Where pregnancy is concerned, it is better to avoid all salad meals when overseas in hot climates and to drink only bottled water, preferably with recognisable branding on it, rather than trust local tap water. You should also be very wary of ice cubes in drinks too for the same reason, as these are sometimes made from questionable tap water. It can often be a good idea to stick to sparkling water for refreshment purposes as the fizz gives a certain guarantee that the water is direct from manufacture, and has not been substituted, as can happen where unscrupulous vendors replace still water products with tap water.

Nutrition for Babies

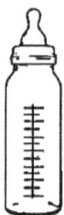

Breast feeding is without doubt the best start in life a baby can have. This is not only because of the high nutritional content of the milk, but more importantly because vital antibodies will be passed on to the infant during the process of feeding. They will protect the baby from many of the viruses its mother has encountered.

Breastfeeding is also beneficial since it enables the mother to use up much of the extra fat deposited during pregnancy. It is important not to eat too much sweet sugary foods at this time though as this could influence the infant in a negative way (for the rest of its life in some cases).

Unfortunately it is not always possible for each new mother to breastfeed. Some new mothers require medication for complications during or after pregnancy and it would be harmful to pass such drugs on to the baby via their milk output. Some mothers also find breastfeeding inconvenient or embarrassing. In the case of both groups, breast milk can be substituted for specific powdered milk.

Whilst such formulas are widely used these days for convenience sake, there can be major disadvantages to them (particularly so where young babies are concerned) in that such formulas rarely meet all the baby's nutritional needs, and do not provide the required antibodies of breast milk for example.

Another disadvantage with powdered milks' can be the sodium (salt) content of them. This can be a particular problem, in that any salt contained in such formulas could make the baby drink more than it needs. Where possible, breast feeding is therefore a far better option for our offspring.

At about six months, it is possible to start weaning the baby (introducing the baby to solids). This is possible because the baby's stomach and enzymes will be developed sufficiently to start more complex digestive processes, though the process of weaning must be done very gradually.

It is important initially to use solid food simply as an addition to the baby's milk feed. It should be offered in a teaspoon measure. Don't worry if it is not accepted; simply try again at a later stage. Once solids are accepted they should be phased in gradually, replacing one feed a day, and so on. A wide choice of commercial products are available for this purpose (in jars and tins), though the most nutritious meals are those made at home in a blender or mashed, i.e. fruit, vegetables, egg etc. Where eggs are used, they should be cooked thoroughly however, to reduce any potential risk of salmonella poisoning (as applies with eggs in respect to pregnancy).

Under no circumstances should newly weaned infants be given adult processed foods to eat at this stage, since their bodies will find it very difficult to deal with the high sodium levels found in these foods.

It is also important to be aware that many of the prepared meals available for infants these days, can also have some degree of salt or sugar in them. Whilst such levels of salt are not likely to cause the baby any harm, like milk substitutes, they are inclined to make a baby rather thirsty. Excessive sugar contents on the other hand are likely to result in an unhealthy craving for sweet food on the baby's part. This could prove a real problem in times to come, especially when the child's teeth develop; also later on in adult life, when a continued craving for sweet foods could lead to obesity and resultant health problems.

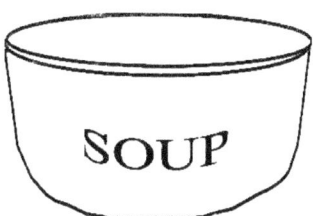

Soups (preferably home made) can be a very nutritious meal for the infant, though in some cases they may clash with the infant's milk feeds. Again as in the case of pregnancy; when preparing chicken and other meats for a small child, it's important to ensure that the meat is cooked thoroughly and that all utensils, blender components, bowls, and plates etc are washed thoroughly.

Also on the subject of safety - when food can be digested in a more solid state, it's important to watch the baby closely, in case they should choke, particularly when diced apple or fish are given as a meal.

How the child develops nutritionally from here on is up to its parents and circumstances, i.e. finance, locality and the time available for food preparation and education.

Nutrition for Children

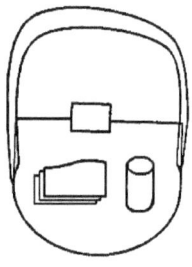

Much will depend upon the family background in respect to nutritional opportunity and circumstances, where balanced meals are concerned. Whilst some children have the opportunity to enjoy nutritious school meals, this does not apply to all and so nutritional responsibility during schooling years still lies very much with the parents both in a physical sense and in terms of nutritional education (which is extremely important).

In some cases (particularly with older children) funding is made available so that children can make their own nutritional provision. In other cases however, children are sent off to school with a packed lunch. Where such foods are provided in a packed lunch format, it's important to vary a child's diet as much as you can, replacing crisps if possible with healthier options, but being realistic. Whilst food education and dietary steering is very important, it is also essential to ensure that the nutrition provided to children is appetising, which usually means tasty and full of colour or flavour.

The snack foods mentioned in the following example, and others on following pages may raise a few eyebrows. Please note that I have stated that such foods should preferably be health orientated variants of the said snacks, i.e. low fat/salt crisps, chocolate, cakes etc low in sugar, and varied, rather than being a constant ingredient in any meal sequence.

The usual format for a packed lunch is as follows - one round of sandwiches (filling to suit); one packet of crisps **(preferably low salt/saturated fat content)**; one item of fruit and a fruit drink of some type **(preferably one with a low sugar content)**. Also as a treat for the child, a bar of chocolate can be included. This meal is in itself quite sufficient if all the items are consumed; sadly this rarely happens with children though, the sandwiches are sometimes discarded and left uneaten either because of distraction or preference.

It is therefore up to the parent to address this problem, both by education, and also by providing a suitable cooked meal at the end of the day.

During the school years it should be ensured that children consume generous amounts of vitamin C rich foods, i.e. fruit and vegetables. These will give the children extra protection against the perpetual onslaught of viruses, carried around the school classrooms and corridors during the winter months (when the heating is on full blast and the children are more confined).

Whilst the children are growing up, it's the parent's responsibility to see they get ample amounts of calcium for their bones (generally found in dairy products). Where a vegetarian lifestyle is chosen, calcium can also be obtained by consuming adequate amounts of nuts, fruit and vegetables. It is possible that as girls grow up they will rebel against dairy products for fear of putting on too much weight.

Where young people do have a reluctance to eat dairy rich foods, they should be advised to maintain a low-fat dairy diet of some type to ensure that they get all the nutrients they require (or to consume more vegetables, fruit and nuts, provided they have a tolerance for these foods).

Nutrition for Teenagers

In the case of girls approaching puberty, it may be necessary to review their diet since their menstrual cycle will begin and their requirements for Iron and B group vitamins will increase tremendously. Again where a rebellion against meat products is in evidence, great care should be taken in explaining the risks and disadvantages of a meat-free, non dairy diet, i.e. the risk of anaemia and the many associated disorders which can result of nutrient deficiency.

Whilst those in this age group should be advised to maintain a wide ranging diet including dairy products where practical (to ensure that they get all the nutrients they require), those choosing to undertake a totally vegetarian diet need to be made aware of other nutritional food options available to them. They may for example be able to get sufficient B group vitamins, Iron etc from fresh vegetable and nut sources alone, but (as with pregnancy), careful supervision by a medical practitioner would be a wise precaution in this situation.

People's dietary needs vary tremendously for each life-stage and are governed by careers (either in a physical, or in many cases, a mental capacity), and also by people's hobbies and interests. As the following groups indicate, there can be a vast difference between people at the same life-stage and their individual requirements.

Where young adults are concerned, much will depend upon whether they have completed their basic schooling, or if they intend to continue academic studies, also if they take an active interest in sports and physical leisure activities.

Students and Clerical Workers

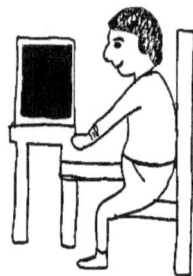

Those choosing to study at school or college, or engage in a clerical career without any intentions of physical labour, need to pay special attention to their diet.

If their diets are unduly balanced in favour of fatty and high carbohydrate foods, those concerned, run the risk of serious health problems in later life. It's often the case that these individuals have a tendency towards snacking and fast foods because their recreational and break times are greatly restricted by their working regimes. Although they are in a high risk health group, they can go a long way to reducing the risks to their health by taking plenty of exercise, by walking or cycling to their place of work or study, for example.

In the case of academic and clerical workers - It is recommended that their diet is made up of fresh fruit and vegetables, lean meat, fish, poultry and eggs. As I've already indicated, this group of people should be careful not to eat too many saturated fats, i.e. dairy produce and fast foods, hamburgers/beef-burgers, pizzas, curry's, chips, etc.

They should also restrict the amount of fried or heavily refined foods (such as white bread and sugar etc) which they consume too, since the energy potential of these types of food are unlikely to be realised and could lead to excessive weight gain or cardio-vascular problems in later life.

The recommended calorie allowance for this group (who undertake little or no exercise) is around 1400 calories. Generally speaking a calorie allowance of around 1800 - 2000 would suit those persons who do undertake some form of exercise during their working or leisure time.

The Manual Labourer / Sports-Person

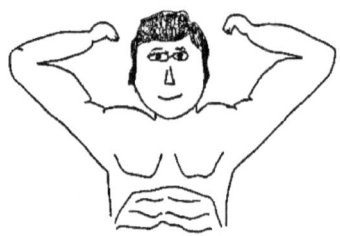

Those persons who have left school to take up a labouring career of some type, or are engaged in sporting pursuits are generally more fortunate in their dietary options. Because of their physical activities, more high calorie foodstuffs can be consumed, (i.e. fats and carbohydrates), though those involved in sport, do have performance to take into account when calculating their dietary needs.

They are also more fortunate, in that unlike their more sedentary counterparts, they are often advised and monitored by their trainers or coaches, in respect to their diets and performance. This being the case, any imbalances, (i.e. weight gain, energy levels etc) are quickly spotted by those watching over them and put right at the earliest opportunity.

Both groups require a high protein intake to combat the excessive wear their bodies will experience. It should be noted however (particularly in the case of sportsmen) that if protein intake is excessive, the body will automatically convert some of it into fuel. If that surplus protein reserve is not used up through activity, it could well be laid down as fat.

Young labouring workers, engaged in hard manual labour (i.e. on building sites etc, where their work involves them lifting, carrying, digging etc) should have a more liberal choice in respect to their diet. In theory they should burn up much of their fat intake (that said, a lot depends upon their metabolism, age, family history etc, just as it does with others within the highlighted groups).

Whilst this group of workers should be able to eat more fat; that does not mean to excess. As with all individuals, too much fatty food will inevitably lead to health issues in many cases, even if we can't see them developing. (Yet again, any of the general dietary options in this document would prove sufficient to maintain such individuals.)

In the case of labouring workers, some choose to take a packed lunch to work with them (as do some children). In many cases nowadays however, such workers tend to use mobile catering or use nearly food outlets to meet their daily dietary needs.

Where such workers do still take a packed lunch, the chocolate bar mentioned in the children's lunch pack would most likely be replaced by a piece of cake (a slightly healthier option if it is home made with quality ingredients and reduced salt, sugar etc). The general calorific allowance for this group is around 2000 - 2500 per day, depending upon gender and after work activities. These guidelines are suitable as people mature into their 20s and 30s, though it should be realised that from 30 onwards (generally speaking) the body has reached its peak of fitness and starts to degenerate. It is therefore essential that a sensible diet regime is established from then on: Failure to observe the basic rules of nutrition from this period may result in serious problems in later life.

Dietary Needs for Middle Age

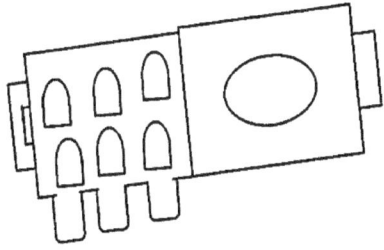

There are few life stage health problems which men encounter, though from middle age it is advisable to regularly monitor the amount of eggs consumed each week, and if necessary cut down on them, if over-consumption is suspected, since they are known to contain high levels of cholesterol, as is true with dairy produce.

Over-consumption of dairy produce (with the exception of the low-fat dairy range) could cause serious cardio-vascular congestion in later life; though this does of course depend upon how physically active people are, and their genetic susceptibility to such problems.

Female Complications

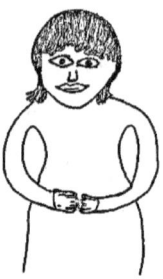

One common condition where women are concerned can be pre-menstrual syndrome P.M.S. Not only can such a condition be very uncomfortable, such conditions can also be extremely disruptive too. Fortunately there are several things that can be done to reduce the effects of P.M.S. It is known for example that increasing the intake of B group vitamins (particularly B6) will (along with exercise), help to reduce the symptoms.

Fresh fruit and vegetables, white meat, fish, and wholemeal bread are strongly recommended; since they contain the B complex nutrients (Iron will also be required at this time of course).

It is known that eating small amounts of such food throughout the day will help.

Such foods as refined sugar, white bread (non-wholemeal), acidic or fatty foods are to be avoided, since bad dietary habits can influence the severity of symptoms.

Women can also encounter problems as a result of the menopause. Much research has been done on the subject and it has been found that vitamin E found in cereals, fruit and vegetables, will be needed at this time. (It apparently prevents the destruction of sex hormones.) As in pre-menstrual syndrome, vitamin B6 has a very important role to play in hormone balance.

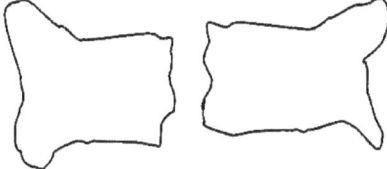

Osteoporosis (a thinning of the bones) is yet another complication which can sometimes occur. This problem is also connected with the female reproductive cycle, since it is in part, caused by a reduction of oestrogen. As well as being one of the female sex hormones, oestrogen is also very much involved with the metabolism of calcium within the female body. Because oestrogen is such an important hormone in the female body, the adrenal glands have been designed to take over its production once the menopause has taken place.

Under normal circumstances, the adrenal glands secrete a specific chemical which travels in the bloodstream to the fatty tissues, where it is converted into oestrogen. Sadly this does not always happen, and so some women can become seriously deficient of oestrogen. In time this can cause a deficiency of calcium within their bodies.

Calcium is a very precious commodity indeed, since it makes up the main part of our skeletal system. Unfortunately calcium is very prone to leaching (i.e. being easily flushed from our bodies) and so we need large quantities to maintain our skeletal systems. That's one of the main reasons we benefit greatly from eating high calcium foods such as milk, dairy produce etc in our earlier years, in order to make our bones good and strong for later life.

As a result of extensive studies into the problem, we now know that through a calcium enriched diet, combined with regular exercise, it is possible to limit, or even reverse the condition in some cases.

Surprising though it may seem, exercise can have a big part to play in respect to relief from such a condition. This is because exercise will stimulate blood supply, which will increase the level of hormones moving round the body, and will likewise help to distribute essential nutrients (including oxygen) to bodily tissue (bones etc).

In respect to specific dietary measures available for the condition, it has been found that cheese and tinned fish, e.g. sardines, have the highest concentrations of calcium. They should therefore be included in a sufferer's weekly meal where possible, though of course excessive cheese intake may be unwise in certain cases, i.e. weight loss, arthritic conditions etc. (Where vegetables are concerned, it has been found that, spinach has the highest calcium content.)

Dietary Needs for Old Age

As old age occurs, both sexes are likely to encounter visual impairment to an equal degree. This is likely to be far less traumatic if the general diet plan as described in this document is adhered to however, especially where plenty of fresh fruit and vegetables have been a regular part of our diet.

SPECIALISED DIETS

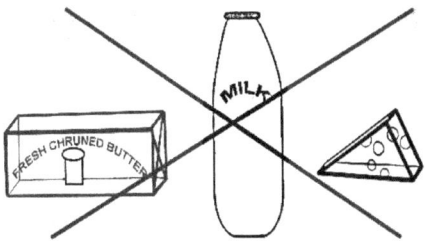

At certain stages in life, metabolic malfunctions can occur and it may be necessary to exclude certain foods completely so as to stabilise or correct a problem. Allergies are one such problem where a person's body reacts sometimes violently against one type of food.

The most common food allergies can be a reaction to dairy produce, nuts or grain (These can occur at any age and for unclear reasons). In such cases, a specific diet will be required, one which will still be nutritious but which excludes the offending foodstuffs concerned.

In certain allergy cases, an even more restricted diet is prescribed, one which is specifically designed to boost the immune system.

In illnesses such as arthritis, migraine, asthma and M.E. a vegetarian diet is strongly recommended, since few vegetables clash with the immune system. Many vegetables contain vitamin E, which as well as being good for the blood and circulation is also anti-inflammatory. On such a diet, it is advisable to exclude citrus fruit, fried foods, potatoes and peppers, as these foods are known to irritate the immune system. Soya milk should be drunk as for the non-dairy diet, preferably on its own, since it is rich in unsaturated fats.

One of the greatest problems in adopting a vegetarian diet - particularly a dairy-free diet, can be the absorption of nutrients, which can be seriously impeded by such diets. They should therefore only be used under medical supervision, or with a qualified dietician's approval.

As I have already indicated, a deficiency in any material component is likely to create a chronic or acute health problem, depending upon the deficient nutrients concerned. Whilst it can be said that artificial supplementation is a way round this problem, it is seldom effective as a main nutrient force in place of those original components which are lost when on a specialised diet.

Those people making dietary adjustments for health reasons should be aware of the many chemical compounds present in modern prepared foodstuffs too. Compounds such as added salt and sugar are to be commonly found in tinned and bottled foods for example.

Sodium and sugar have always been used to preserve foodstuffs and it should be realised that these two additives can prove very detrimental in conditions such as obesity and heart complaints. It is therefore, much better to eat fresh produce (rather than commercial mass produced produce) when dietary adjustments or restrictions are necessary.

Other factors to take into consideration are the food's history and its subsequent preparation, both of which can make a considerable difference to the nutritional value of the foodstuffs consumed.

DIGESTIVE DISORDERS

Another area where dietary caution applies is in respect to stomach complaints; the most common of these being Hiatus Hernias, Ulcers, Crohns Disease, Irritable Bowel Syndrome, Diabetes, Diverticulitis: also Diarrhoea, and sickness of course. All can be very unpleasant, and require urgent medical attention on occasion. It is often possible to manage such conditions with dietary measures however, as I will outline shortly.

In the case of the first conditions mentioned, long-term adjustments will often be required, in terms of dietary intake (the timing of meals/type of meal), and emotional behaviour (stress responses), also in respect to physical posture in the case of hiatus hernia and stomach ulcers.

Hiatus Hernia

Among the most common of these conditions is the Hiatus Hernia. This particular condition is generally caused by a defect, or damage to a small valve in the upper stomach. When we eat fatty foods we use acids from our stomach to break the fat down. Under normal circumstances the valve at the top of our stomach shuts to seal in any food we are digesting, so that the acid and other digestive juices can get to work. If for some reason the valve at the top of our stomach is damaged then these acids will be allowed, along with any partially digested foods, to rise back up into our gullet (a condition called acid reflux).

      Whereas our stomach is designed to cope with our digestive juices, the gullet is not, and so it soon gets very sore, which makes swallowing food very difficult. This frequently leads to feelings of nausea and pain, where the acids in the digestive juices, burn into the lining of the gullet, or sometimes, gasses build up within the stomach itself and are unable to escape (a condition called wind or heartburn) which makes us feel very bloated. As the name heartburn indicates, this can be, and frequently is, a very painful condition.

In respect to treating the condition, much will depend upon our life-stage and lifestyle and so it is not possible to set out a specific diet to treat the condition, other than to suggest a reduction in consumption of fatty foods.

In the past it was recommended that people suffering acidity problems avoid eating fatty foods altogether, this has now been acknowledged as a mistake because we need a small degree of fats in our diet to give us energy, both in a physical sense, and a mental one.

Following much research it has been discovered that spicy and fried foods in particular will aggravate the condition. They should therefore be avoided wherever possible when symptoms of indigestion present themselves. Other than that, a normal diet should be maintained as much as possible, according to our life-stage and lifestyle, whilst possibly lowering out fat intake, should this prove helpful to our condition.

Those with this condition should also take into account the guidelines in this book about the consequences of eating too much fat, i.e. too many packets of crisps, ready meals etc, so as not to aggravate their condition.

It is also important to realise that with a hiatus hernia, posture plays an important part in respect to the condition, particularly in respect to mealtimes. With such a condition it is inadvisable to take breakfast in bed for example, also bending down soon after a meal will aggravate the condition, as the acids will be drawn back up into the gullet in both cases.

Although many antacids and medicines are available in respect to acid related illnesses, they will not provide long-term relief and so those issues I've just mentioned will need to be addressed.

Stomach Ulcers

Where stomach ulcers occur they are often (although not exclusively, as it is known that certain types of medicine can cause them too) closely associated with stress and so lifestyle management and reactionary review (amendments to our emotional stress responses) can play a very big part in the treatment of the condition.

When people are stressed, their bodies pump extra digestive juices into their stomach so that any food will be digested quickly. In the past this would have been beneficial since it would have made us lighter and more able to flee any threatening physical situation if necessary. These days however, we live in a very different world; our stresses originate not from physical threats, but from mental ones.

Nowadays we are under constant stress because of our modern working practices, and lifestyles generally.

Sadly our bodies are not able to adjust to this modern lifestyle; when we are stressed, they respond just the same as they have always done, in that they secrete large amounts of acid. Very often our stomachs are empty at the time and so the excess amounts of acids are floating about in our stomachs looking for some material to break down.

Although our digestive systems are designed to deal with acid, they are meant to contain food when the acid is present and this normally takes the brunt of chemical action in respect to the acid.

When our stomachs are empty, it is our stomach linings themselves which take the full force of the acids and so after a while of perpetual acid onslaught, they break down in places making ulcerations, which if left untreated will cause abdominal bleeding.

In respect to this condition, it has been found that eating small amounts of carbohydrates (plain biscuits) regularly during the day, together with milk, will help to mop up any excess acid. (Milk in itself is particularly good in respect to neutralising the effects of acid.) As with a hiatus hernia, it is advisable to avoid fried and spicy foods, and drinks such as coffee whenever possible.

The principle treatment in respect to this condition generally relates to lifestyle adjustment however, both in respect to the way we deal with stress, and also, in respect to eating regularly. It has been found that many ulcer sufferers are people who are on the go for most of the day, who skip breakfast, and fail to eat at regular times. All of these things are known to be bad for our digestion.

The eating of regular meals, sticking to a basic food diet (as outlined in some of the specialised diet pages), the avoidance of spicy/fried foods and coffee wherever possible, resting after a meal, and of course, amending our personal stress loading are all important. Such actions will all affect the severity of symptoms in a positive way. Certain types of medication may also be required, either on a short or long-term basis too.

Irritable Bowel Syndrome/ Crohnes Disease

In some cases, as with Irritable Bowel Syndrome, a whole host of inexplicable reasons can trigger such conditions, i.e. an allergy, stress etc, and it can be very difficult to pin down an exact cause. One way to limit the effects of this condition however; can be to keep a food and general diary, and to link it with symptoms when they occur. This can often help to identify foods or situations which trigger such conditions.

<u>Diverticulitis</u>

Another common digestive condition can be Diverticulitis, where the lower stomach develops small bulging sacs. It's a situation which seems to occur more frequently in older people (from middle age onwards). These bulging sacs can sometimes trap food and become infected, leading to great pain and possible complications.
     In respect to the treatment for Diverticulitis; it is known that consuming too much rough fibre, nuts, cereal bran etc can aggravate the condition, therefore softer sources of fibre should be consumed instead. It is particularly important to takes such steps during episodes of illness. It is also a bad idea to consume too many stodgy foods on a regular basis too, since such foods can aggravate the condition.

Diabetes

Another extremely serious digestive condition, comes in the form of diabetes. If left untreated/unmanaged, diabetes can cause blindness, nervous collapse, hear attacks, strokes, loss of limbs and a whole host of other very serious life threatening conditions. Diabetes must therefore always be taken seriously should it be discovered in someone.

Sadly this particularly nasty illness is becoming increasingly common these days thanks in part to our over-consumption of sweet and heavily processed foods. (Genetic pre-disposition can and does also play a part in illness susceptibility too of course.)

There are basically two forms of diabetes; Type 1 and type 2. Whilst both are very serious, type 1 is far more so. That s because with this version of the illness, an essential chemical (insulin) which helps us is turn glucose sugar into energy does not get produced by the pancreas as it should do. Because of this, sufferers of this condition can be virtually poisoned by an overload of unusable energy.

In the case of type 1 diabetes, sufferers of this type generally have to inject themselves regularly with insulin in order to overcome this situation, in order to make their bodies work as they should.

With type two diabetes (where insulin function does not work very well), dietary management can often be enough to keep the condition in check, though medical monitoring is still required. The most alarming thing about this condition however can be its ability to remain unnoticed until symptoms are well advanced.

Fortunately the medical profession is always on the lookout for this nasty illness and it is often during routine tests that the condition is picked up. In the case of both types of diabetes, a radical change in diet will be required to keep the condition in check. There are a whole host of foods which should be avoided.

The most important foods to avoid when suffering diabetes are as follows: i.e. sugary sweets, cakes and pastry, fatty meats, sweetened fruit drinks; full fat milk/dairy produce, dried fruits such as apricots, dates raisins etc, white bread, chips and other fried foods.

    Not only do these foods contain too much sugar for diabetics to handle, they can also bring about serious weight gain which can also cause problems in respect to the condition. Low fat dairy produce and some types of fruit can be beneficial under supervision. It is also important to ensure that an adequate amount of fluids are consumed too, as dehydration is always a risk in respect to diabetes.

    Whilst it is a very complex and serious condition, with careful dietary management and medical supervision it is possible to live a normal life even with this condition, by sticking to plain and simple foods, and by taking regular exercise. It is now believed that if those with type 2 diabetes abstain from problem foods at an early stage of the illness, it can sometimes be possible to overcome this disease, though research is still going on into this possibility.

Diarrhoea and Sickness

Digestive upsets are another area where care needs to be taken too. They can of course take many forms, diarrhoea and sickness being two clear examples.

These last two conditions can often relate to a form of infection, either as a result of something we have eaten, inhaled or touched. Sadly a great many viruses and bacteria target the digestive tract and are likely to cause a great deal of discomfort.

In both cases where digestive illnesses occur, food ingestion will be a very difficult task, either from the point of keeping it down, or absorbing the nutrients we have ingested. When trying to cope with both these situations, it's very important not to overload the digestive tract and so small meals are required in both cases, either in liquid form, i.e. soups etc, or in solid form i.e. dry biscuits/toast etc. As individuals, we each have different tastes and some foods will be more appetising than others. With both cases its best to keep meals simple at first.

In respect to diarrhoea conditions, it's often best to stop eating for a while until the bacteria have cleared our system. In such cases it is essential that we drink fluids on a regular basis however, since dehydration is a very common occurrence with this situation.

In all cases of digestive disorders, it is very important to seek medical advice if symptoms are very severe, or last for more than 48 hours (particularly where children are concerned).

DAIRY/LACTOSE FREE/ DIET

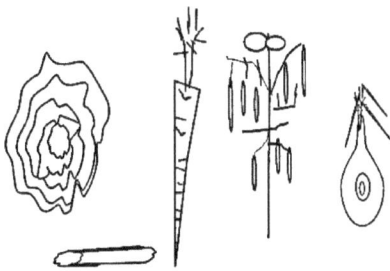

(Those with health problems, intolerances and digestive issues should beware in respect to some of these food examples below and on the next pages, taking care to avoid certain acid foods and fruit juices of the type mentioned below, along with those foods known to cause allergic reaction. **(Please choose suitable alternatives instead.)** Where pastry based pies are mentioned below, it is assumed that vegetarian materials will be used **(Please see internet, for more details and range of pastry options available)**.

SUGGESTED BEVERAGE OPTIONS:

Fruit juices, soy milk **(in moderation)**, mineral water, tea (preferably herb or fruit).

SUGGESTED BREAKFAST OPTIONS:

A bowl of breakfast cereal with soy milk, **(in small quantity)**. /An item or items of fruit.

Toast with margarine, egg or jam.

SUGGESTED LUNCH OPTIONS:

A bread roll with various fillings **(margarine instead of butter)**, i.e. salad, ham, chicken, egg, **(preferably removing fat from any ham/ and removing chicken skin before consumption)**.

Baked potato with fillings, (as for roll).

Soup or beans on toast.

SUGGESTED EVENING MEAL OPTIONS:

Boiled potatoes, greens, lambs liver or kidney.

Shepherds pie with green vegetables.

Salad with pasta, nuts, fruit, fish or chicken. / sardines on toast.

Steak and kidney/chicken pie **(using dairy-free pastry ingredients)** with potatoes and vegetables.

Spaghetti bolognaise, **(preferably home made with good quality ingredients)**.

SUGGESTED SWEET OPTIONS: (if required).

Fresh fruit.

Fruit pie, ie homemade apple etc **(using dairy-Free pastry ingredients)**.

Jelly.

LOW CALORIE DIET SUITABLE FOR HEART COMPLAINTS AND WEIGHT PROBLEMS

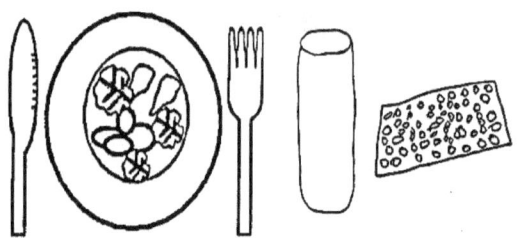

SUGGESTED BEVERAGE OPTIONS:

Skimmed or soy milk, unsweetened fruit juice, mineral water, and herb tea.

SUGGESTED BREAKFAST OPTIONS:

Half grapefruit.

One small bowl of breakfast cereal with either soy milk **(in moderation)** or skimmed milk, (artificial sweetener if required).

One piece of crisp bread with low fat spread with apricot (dried rather than tinned).
One piece of toast with low fat spread with tinned fish, e.g. sardines.

SUGGESTED LUNCH OPTIONS:

Wholemeal bread roll with tinned fish filling or grated carrot, one cup of vegetable soup, wholemeal sandwich with lettuce/tomato filling, beans on toast.

SUGGESTED MAIN MEAL OPTIONS:

Salad with pasta, lean meat or fish, grated raw carrots, peanuts (non-salted), onion.

Boiled potatoes, green vegetables, lean boiled ham.

Salad with rice, chicken, peanuts, grated carrot.

Besides these typical examples there are an infinite range of low-calorie food combinations which can be tried and consumed to suit our particular taste.

PERSONAL CIRCUMSTANCES

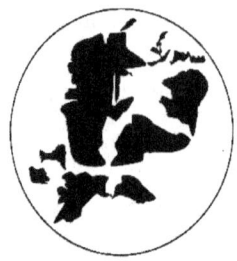

Diets vary considerably from country to country and so by looking at each nation's nutritional habits, we are able to get comprehensive data as to which foods are of most benefit to us. It has been found for example that fishing nations i.e. the Japanese, Norwegian, Icelandic, and some Far Eastern nations seem to live the healthiest of lives, though as a result of western influence (i.e. fast food restaurants) many Asian nations are sadly catching us up in respect to health problems.

    A great many countries in the east thrive on basic rice dishes, whilst others in the Far East prefer bread based meals. In the Mediterranean salad based foods are preferable. In the West we eat a great many foods, most of which are heavily refined.

    Diets can also vary tremendously,

depending upon which class system and district we are born into. We are from birth programmed to live within such systems and regimes. In the early stages of life we are very much dependent upon our parents for our dietary guidance. They in turn are very much influenced by their social status. **(I refer not so much to modern England, but to some Asian and African regions for example, where the class system still remains and many items of food are in short supply.)**

Many children grow up in such societies with poor educational facilities and with a set lifestyle, i.e. as a farm labourer, having to grow their own produce in order to survive. They know and adhere to a healthy dietary regime far better than those of the richer classes.

More often than not they live on a very basic diet, balanced equally with fresh green vegetables, carbohydrates and some animal proteins. The more affluent groups of such societies however, tend to feast on highly-refined carbohydrates, and high-proportioned fatty foods, whilst taking very little physical exercise (and with no dietary planning whatsoever). This can lead to chronic illness, varying from dowager's hump to atherosclerosis.

Whereas the labouring classes stick to basic nutritional food, the affluent classes are more interested in presentation and taste, being in a better position to afford the trimmings and looking upon meals as a social occasion, rather than an opportunity to restock their bodies with fuel. We in the west have for the most part fallen into the same trap though for very different reasons (a breakdown of the family unit for instance).

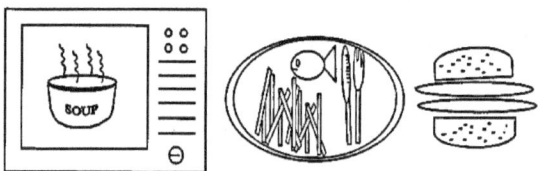

In the Western world we now have many single-parent families, with each parent struggling to provide for their children as best they can. Parents who find themselves in such a position are often forced to find employment at the earliest opportunity in order to make ends meet.

The knock on effect of this is that the child's nutritional education and programming for the future can sometimes go astray. Because money is short and time is even shorter, the parent is often forced to opt for convenience foods as a suitable meal for their dependants and themselves. Sadly few single parents get the opportunity to redress the balance, since they don't have time to grow or prepare the genuinely nutritious foods that are available to them: This gives rise to a fast-food society.

Being only too well aware of this situation, the various manufacturers, jostle enthusiastically for prime selling position, in what is now a huge market.

Cunningly they tempt us with brightly coloured packaging, and large advertising campaigns. The food itself is often laced with potent artificial colouring, flavourings, preservatives and other matter (i.e. standard packets of crisps, etc). None of these are good for us if consumed in large doses, and yet these days such foods often go to make up a substantial part of our diet.

ORGANIC OR MASS-PRODUCED?

This question is one which all of us will face at some stage or other, particularly when we have been ill and suffered from one of the illnesses mentioned in this book.

More often than not, we have been so short of time that we have had no option other than to opt for convenience foods. Because the food has been produced elsewhere, we have no idea as regards the nutrient quality of what we are buying. As I've already indicated, in the case of vegetables for example (which should be high in nutrients), much will depend upon the type of soil they are grown in.

In some cases, vegetables will have been grown traditionally/organically, in well-managed soil, using a traditional rotation system. (Under this system, a series of nutrient replacing plant crops will have been rotated in sequence, on land which is free of pesticides, that has been regularly manured, and has been periodically rested.) More often than not however, the crops we buy will have been produced intensively, in soil which has been in constant use, using high yield fertilisers.

Sadly these two very different forms of production can make a considerable difference in respect to the nutritional value of any crops that are produced, both in terms of nutritional value, and also, just importantly, their cost. In respect to the options of organic or "mass produced," that is where mass producers win hands down, in that by producing on a large scale, they are able to keep their costs down, and can meet the requirements of large wholesalers such as supermarkets, fast food producers etc in respect to high volume and constant supply.

Organic food producers often work on a much smaller scale. Their crops and livestock can take a lot longer to produce, compared to those produced by their more commercially minded mass producing competitors. This is principally because an organic producer will be using natural organisms and seasonal conditions to produce their crops, rather than fast producing chemical compounds. This will therefore inevitably make any such crops or livestock produced organically, that more expensive to produce and to buy.

As with most things, as consumers we get what we pay for, and this is certainly true where vegetables and fruit are concerned. Whilst organic produce is far more expensive than the mass-produced alternative, the quality and nutritious value of such crops, grossly exceeds that of the more common mass produced alternative in a good many cases. On a health basis, we should therefore aim to buy organic foods wherever possible. Not only are they free from commercial chemicals, they are also monitored regularly as to their purity, with the soils that produce them, likewise being subject to regular testing in most cases. Sadly however, it is the commercial mass-market producers which have the upper hand these days, due mainly to commercial factors beyond our control.

During the past few decades a great many changes have occurred in respect to our agricultural industry and food production generally, changes which unfortunately have made a big difference to the quality of the food we now eat.

Because we have moved away from basic farming and into intensive agriculture, our food is grown in bulk and inevitably stored, or in some cases has come from abroad. Both these practices undermine the nutritional value of the produce. From the minute a crop is harvested, it starts to deteriorate both physically and nutritionally. It is therefore, imperative that we eat the food as soon as we can; this seldom happens however.

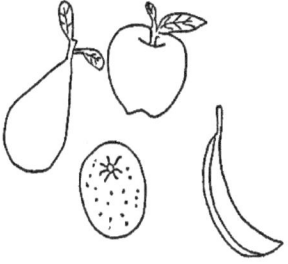

More often than not the produce we are offered is days old rather than hours, as it used to be. In the case of fruit and tomatoes, they are picked before they are ripe, to allow for transportation. Although people may not realise it, this is a practice which greatly undermines the nutritional value of the products concerned, because it denies them the natural sunlight they needs to ripen properly.

Because of premature picking, many fruits can often be deficient in vitamin C. (It is during the ripening process that vitamin C normally reaches its peak). A similar situation applies to vegetables as well. By the time many of them reach the kitchen they too can be very low in respect to some nutrients. It is therefore very important to realise this when cooking them - preferably by boiling them on a low heat, for as short a time as possible.

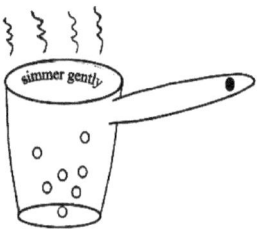

Whilst we would all be so much healthier if we grew our own produce, for most of us this is no longer possible, either from the point of time and energy expended that would be needed to grow them, or the land we would need to set aside for such a project.

Our lifestyles and work patterns have changed to such a degree over recent years that it is no longer feasible for us to grow our own produce in most cases. Unfortunately, because of our hectic lifestyles, we are now very much at the mercy of those who choose to produce food on our behalf.

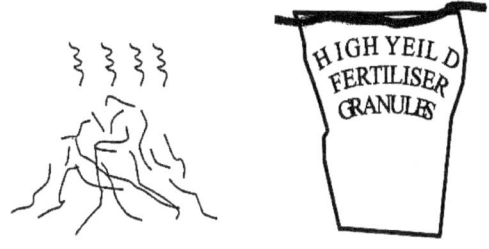

Besides our lifestyles changing, agricultural practices have changed too. These days, fewer of our farmers are keeping livestock for example, because of this, natural fertilisers which were once freely available for both domestic and market gardeners to use to enrich their soil, are now very hard to come by.

They have by and large been replaced by chemical compounds of one form or another, which nutritionally and environmentally speaking, do us no good in the long term, because they make food develop too quickly.

Although speedy food production might seem advantageous, sadly this is far from the truth, for it means that the crops concerned have less time to absorb the very vitamins and minerals we are eating them for. The environmental impact of such crops can also be disastrous for the environment as well.

Many of the chemical fertilisers used to make the crops grow are very prone to leaching (being carried away by rain to our watercourses) and also liable to drifting during application.

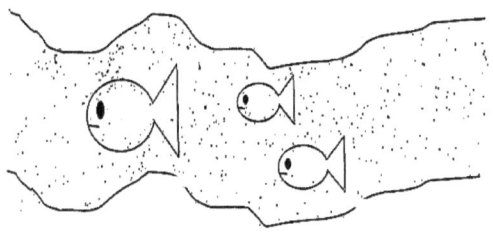

Nitrogen is a prime example where our interference in respect to chemicals has cost us dearly; you have only to look at our rivers to see this. In some cases the ecological balance of our rivers has been severely disturbed where high nitrogen fertilisers have contaminated the watercourse.

In extreme cases such contamination can make the river weed and algae grow to such a degree that they block out the sun's rays and turn the watercourse stagnant. As a result of this, many of the plants and creatures living in the water are likely to die through lack of oxygen. Such incidents were unlikely to occur in the past, because we were using more natural, less concentrated nutrients (just as organic farmers still do).

European subsidies and the world markets do indeed have a formidable case to answer in respect to the environment. Because of mass producing competition, these days, farmers have to think big and produce their products quickly if they are to survive, and this is where the problem lies. They are after all the custodians of our countryside, and so when they are under pressure we all suffer, either from an environmental, or most importantly, a nutritional perspective.

It's a sad fact, but a great deal of damage has been done to our environment because of modern agricultural methods (the overproduction of corn being a prime example). Farmers have been under pressure to get maximum yields from each acre they own (often at the expense of our wildlife).

In many cases our native wildlife has been starved out of the countryside because of a lack of insect food; or nesting and living quarters; caused by the grubbing out of hedges and overuse of pesticides and herbicides. The plight of this country's wildlife is now desperate; indeed some species are in fact facing extinction as a result of our modern farming methods.

Although we cannot turn the clock back, we should consider the cost to ourselves and the environment when buying our food, in respect to the way our foodstuffs are produced.

Through our purchasing power we can at least have some influence upon those who grow our food so that they behave more responsibly in respect to producing it.

Intensive poultry farming and genetically modified foods are a prime example were we as buyers can have great influence. If we don't buy foods of this type then the producers will be forced to change their methods of production to suit our requirements. In some aspects of food production we have less control however, and so it is up to us to make the most of that produce put before us (i.e. supermarket produce for example). Where possible, support the small local producer who sticks to traditional methods of production.

PROBLEM FOODS

As the title of this chapter clearly indicates, not all food is good for us even though it may have some redeeming features in respect to convenience, or palatability. Despite these apparent virtues, the over consumption of some of these foods can have very negative consequences for us if we are not careful with them.

To make things worse for us as consumers, the classification of such foods varies tremendously according to scientific research/food preparation and processing methods. Advice on good and bad foods changes frequently, almost on a daily basis.

A food which is classified as good for us one day can be labelled as bad a few weeks later or vice versa. Dairy produce, eggs and saturated fats are prime examples of this.

A short while ago dairy produce and eggs were negatively implicated in respect to heart conditions and so many people stopped eating them thinking they were doing themselves some harm eating them.

We have now been told that high quality dairy products and saturated fats are good for us in moderation, as can be the case with wine and chocolate for example). Refined sugar and processed meats are on the current hit list as far as negative foods are concerned. **It is certainly true that all these foods can harm us if consumed too often and in too high a quantity**, but in most cases, for the average person, they do little or no harm when consumed occasionally and in very small amounts.

Where food processing is concerned, this is a very scientific area and we are very much at the mercy of those who oversee such processes and monitor their effects for nutritional purpose.

For a very long time there has been serious concern raised in respect to processed cooking methods, particularly where corn oils are concerned in respect to processed cake and pastry products, margarines etc. There are also serious concerns in respect to processed meats too. In both of these cases it has been found that the properties of such foods can change during the cooking/manufacturing process, whereby harmful elements can be created simply by heating these foods in a certain way.

As well as these two examples of problem foods, there are also those foods which contain wholly natural elements too, foods such as animal products, (particularly meats such as ham and lamb), and cooked pastries in respect to fruit and meat pies, quiches etc. These are both known to be high in saturated fats or calories, also crisps and processed ready meals, i.e. burgers, kebabs (most ready meals in fact).

The main thing to realise about these foods however, is that for a healthy individual, **(if consumed occasionally and in small quantities)** as with the other foods already mentioned in this chapter, they are likely to do us little harm.

It is generally when problem foods become the main part of our diet that they become a serious health risk. Ideally we should aim to eat healthier alternatives wherever possible. Such foods do however cost considerably more and are not so readily available in many cases.

Another issue with meats and some

dairy produce can be shelf life too. As I have indicated in the pregnancy section of this guide, it is essential that we adhere to any, "use by" dates found on packaging if we are to avoid unpleasant illnesses which can arise as a result of bacterial infection. It is also very important to keep such foods at the right temperature too. Where foods are chilled we must keep them chilled; likewise with frozen foods. Where some food is left at room temperature, we often have but a few hours to consume it before it will go off. This especially applies to cooked foods at catering functions for example.

BUYER BEWARE

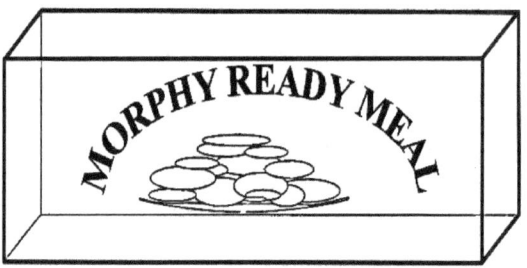

In recent years healthy eating has become very big business, and many supposedly low fat products are now available to us through supermarket and retail outlets, in the form of ready made convenience meals and snacks.

Regrettably many of these products have been found to be no better than their standard counterparts, since they are still reliant upon preservatives, i.e. sugars and salts for extended shelf life. They cannot therefore be recommended as part of a healthy diet. Where possible fresh foods are still the best option in most cases. It's not all doom and gloom however.

Following much publicity about this potential problem, most food producers these days are working hard to reduce such ingredients in our foods, in an attempt to make such meals healthier. Ready meals, dairy produce and fried snack products such as crisps, and biscuit products etc are a prime examples of this, in that there have been considerable improvements in respect to their fat and sodium contents: It is now genuinely possible to buy low fat and sodium products; the same applies to the soft drinks industry too, in that they likewise are working very hard to make previously unhealthy soft drinks more health, reformulating them in a positive way so that we can still enjoy them without them being a potential problem for some people.

      Another area where major advances have been made is that of food supplements, which are now widely available in many formats, namely, oils, tablets, capsules or powders. It is important to acknowledge their potency; they should in the main be used under supervision, since an overdose of any one substance could bring about serious illness. It is therefore a good idea to consult a dietician or doctor before embarking upon any form of supplement. They can however, play an important part in restoring nutritional balance in certain cases, and do therefore have a role to play in the scheme of things.

Besides mainstream vitamin/mineral supplements, there are also a wide range of herbal supplements of various kinds available too, such as Garlic, Aloe Vera, St John's Wort, Echinacia, Ginko Biloba etc; all offering specific remedial properties.

Whilst many herbal and homeopathic remedies may offer hope, and indeed some relief (where specific conditions are concerned), or are taken in a preventative capacity, they cannot necessarily be relied upon as effective. Sadly such product supplements are relatively new to the marketplace and it will be a long time before such compounds/products can be wholly verified as effective.

It can also be the case (especially with St John's wort) that natural based plant and animal products can interact in a negative way with any prescribed medicines, making pre-existing conditions worse, or creating new health complications in some cases.

When intending to take natural based

plant and animal products (or nutritional supplements), it is therefore essential to inform your medical practitioner prior to taking such supplements, especially so where pre-existing conditions are concerned, or where treatment medications have been prescribed.

In respect to general supplements (vitamins and minerals etc), it should also be taken into account that a wide variety of food products now available on our supermarket shelves have been fortified by refined nutrients.

Such items as breakfast cereals, fruit drinks, biscuits and other baked products are often fortified by chemical compounds to replace some of the goodness which has been lost during their manufacture. It is therefore possible that we are in fact getting a large amount of any one nutrient (albeit in an artificial form) and do not need a supplement.

As with all supplements (as I've already indicated), where possible it's best to consult a competent dietician or physician before commencing a course of such supplements.

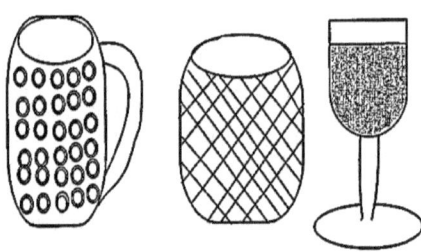

Alcoholic Drinks

Another area where "Buyer Beware" applies is in respect to alcohol. Whilst in some cases, a small amount of alcohol may appear to be of benefit to us emotionally, in helping us to relax, in making us more confident with others etc, sadly there is also a potential downside to alcohol too.

    It is important to note that some recent research seems to indicate that even the smallest amount of alcohol can be harmful to us in a physical context (in respect to our essential organs i.e. our liver etc). The latest research also seems to indicate that consuming any alcohol puts at a greater risk or developing cancer too). As with many others foods items (i.e. meats, dairy products etc), where negative evidence has been found in respect to these foods, other research can likewise be found that contradicts such findings. With alcohol it is therefore, as already stated, very much a "buyer beware" situation until compelling and comprehensive evidence comes to light which will totally confirm or dismiss any negative repercussions in respect to consuming alcohol of all types.

For some, alcoholic dependence can also prove to be a problem when we rely upon alcohol too much to support us emotionally too. Careful self restraint and willpower is therefore needed where alcohol is concerned.

Where alcoholic drinks are deemed to have any benefit to us, it is in respect to the natural fruit or grain constituents in any such drinks. It's often surprising just how many nutrients can be found in many types of alcoholic beverages, particularly wines and beers. In the case of wines, they are known to contain important vitamins, minerals and other nutritious antioxidant components; whilst beer is thought by some to have merit due to its high yeast and vitamin content. As previously stated however, it is important to realise that whilst to some it may appear beneficial or harmless to consume alcohol occasionally and in moderate amounts, the reverse is most definitely true if consumed to excess. The proof of this can be evident in the term "Alcohol Poisoning." This very real and common condition just proves how dangerous it can be to drink too much.

In respect to the damage we could be doing to ourselves; a lot depends upon whether we drink large amounts at a time and on a regular basis (i.e. every day), if we consume the alcohol with food (which can reduce its effects to a degree); if we are male or female, our physical size and whether we are regular consumers of alcohol.

The emotional effects alcohol has upon us also have to be taken into account too.

All these factors will have a bearing upon the effects alcohol will have on us when we drink it. Common sense is therefore crucial when it comes to drinking alcohol, both for our own sake and for others.

We also need to ask ourselves the following questions and know the answers to these two very important questions, i.e. -

Does alcohol make us reckless which will put us and others in danger?

Does alcohol make us aggressive?

Most of us have a pattern of behaviour which applies if we've been drinking. Where we genuinely benefit from alcohol consumption, it's important to use that pattern to our advantage as I indicated in the first paragraph of this chapter. If however we generally experience negative repercussions from our drinking alcohol, it's important to take steps to prevent any harmful patterns from occurring, either by not drinking at all, or by having a minder on hand to help us control our drinking when we are out socially or at home for example; by doing these things, alcohol cannot control us so easily or damage us.

VITAMIN AND MINERAL INDEX

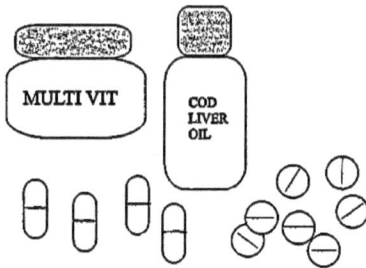

Whilst the aim of this guide is to encourage healthy eating, it has to be acknowledged that there are certain cases where supplements are necessary and so I will summarise those in common usage and explain their functions in the following section –

MINERALS.

IRON - Usually available in tablet or powder form, or in serious cases of deficiency, by way of injection. It is used mainly in cases of anaemia and is often prescribed to supplement losses of iron during pregnancy and the female cycle. The natural alternative sources are meat and vegetables.

CALCIUM/PHOSPHORUS - Supplements are available in various formats and used to reinforce the skeletal (calcium) or neurological system (phosphorus). Calcium/Phosphorus are found mainly in dairy produce and can therefore become deficient where dairy produce is deemed unsuitable for consumption.

SODIUM/POTASSIUM - are tissue salts used to balance fluid levels within the body and are usually given as a supplement in cases of dehydration. (They occur naturally in most foods.)

TRACE ELEMENTS

IODINE - comes usually in tablet or salt form and is given to help glandular/hormonal functions, and primarily for the thyroid gland, which is largely responsible for our metabolism. Iodine occurs naturally in dairy produce, vegetables and seafood.

SELENIUM - also comes either in tablet or salt form, and is sometimes recommended along with iron. Selenium is important for the metabolism of red blood cells and occurs naturally in most foods.

ZINC - is most often available in tablet form, and is very important to the immune system. Supplementation is frequently recommended during illness, being particularly beneficial where colds and flu type symptoms persist, though it is best to stick to the recommended dosage, as an overdose can cause other illness such as digestive tract damage. Zinc is found naturally in most foods.

VITAMINS

As a group vitamins are by far the most common supplement and are available in many forms:

VITAMIN A - (retinol) plays a major role in the health of our external body tissue i.e. our hair, skin and nails, and also the efficiency of our eyesight. Vitamin A occurs naturally in fish oils, dairy produce, fruit and vegetables (carrots in particular).

VITAMIN B Group is made up of at least nine different vitamins. They deal mainly with the metabolism of carbohydrates and blood composition. They are often recommended in cases of anaemia and malnourishment, also during the female cycle and pregnancy. They occur naturally in cereals, fruit, vegetables, meat and dairy produce.

The most common vitamins in this group are as follows –

B.1 (Thiamin).

B.2 (Riboflavin).

B.6

B.12

FOLIC ACID (which together are recommended during pregnancy).

VITAMIN C - is also widely available in many forms and known to be essential for the development of soft body tissue (Vitamin

C is thought to boost the immune system). By far the most common sources are fresh fruit and vegetables. Again as with Zinc, a degree of caution should be applied as eating too many acid rich foods can damage the lining of the stomach.

VITAMIN D - is also found in a wide variety of formats (the most common form of supplement being through fish oil capsules). Vitamin D can be found naturally in fresh fish, dairy produce, margarine and vegetable oils and is known to be essential for the metabolism of calcium.

As I have previously stated, all the above nutrients are available in a refined form, either from our local chemist or health food shop. It is however, important to realise that they are in effect medicines, there to restore nutritional imbalance when illness occurs, or to prevent illness. They are not to be taken without some form of supervision - especially in tablet form - since in such concentrated forms they could damage the liver.

The fish and primrose oils are probably the safest and can prove beneficial where illnesses such as arthritis have been diagnosed.

    Occasionally protein supplements will be recommended, usually following a serious illness or during training for a major athletic or sporting event.

    It is important to realise that used unnecessarily, such extra protein will in fact be laid down as fat and would prove counter-productive in the long run - likewise in the case of glucose supplements which are often given during or after illness.

VEGETARIAN DIETS

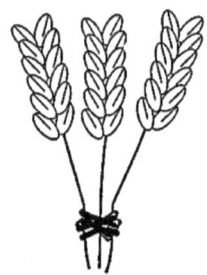

Vegetarian diets are becoming more and more common these days and for a very wide range of reasons. In some cases people feel guilty about the livestock reared and slaughtered to provide us with food.

In other cases people choose not to eat meat because of the numerous health scares associated with meat/dairy produce (BSE, salmonella, the perceived risks of cancer, chemical poisoning, circulatory disorders i.e. heart attacks and strokes etc), widely publicised in the media these days.

Whilst vegetarian principles are certainly beneficial to most livestock, they are not necessarily beneficial for those undertaking such diets - especially those who opt for a full vegan diet, without any dairy produce at all.

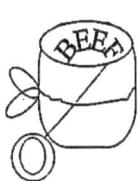 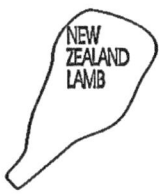 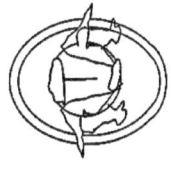

As the early pages of this booklet show, dairy/meat products should play an essential part in our dietary intake (particularly for women). Omitting such valuable sources of nutrition from our diet can result in serious long-term health disorders, such as osteoporosis for example.

It can be argued that vegetable matter provides sufficient minerals and vitamins to satisfy our needs, but this is only true if the foodstuffs are grown in ideal conditions (i.e. well manured ground, totally free of pesticides and preservatives and eaten within a few hours of harvesting). In the normal course of events these criteria are almost impossible to guarantee.

Another common problem which can occur in vegetarian diets is that of anaemia, caused through a deficiency of the many B group vitamins, most commonly found in meat products. They are largely required for our metabolism and blood composition and nervous system and so a deficiency in any one of these components can have very serious consequences in the long term.

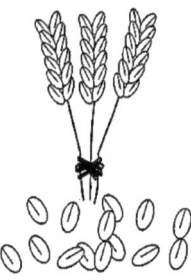

It can again be argued that those vital nutrients can be obtained through consuming various types of grain, but again, as with the minerals I mentioned just now, they are subject to the same criteria of source and method of production.

Another very common problem with a high cereal intake can be nutrient lockup. Regrettably, it's a proven fact that a high intake of fibre can greatly impede nutrient intake - especially major nutrients such as calcium, iron and zinc.

Although it is indeed admirable to consider any livestock caught up in our food chain, it is not necessarily beneficial to our own health to abstain from meat altogether. It is far better to reduce our meat intake rather than stop eating meat completely. By doing so it's possible to strike a sensible balance between satisfying our nutritional needs and reducing the number of animals required for our direct consumption.

Whilst it is clearly beneficial to maintain a reasonable level of meat and dairy consumption, ultimately whether or not we do is a matter of personal conscience at the end of the day. As a result of much publicity in respect to animal welfare there are an increasing number who choose not to eat meat these days. As I've indicated however, an element of risk clearly exists where meat and dairy produce are wholly excluded from our diet, therefore a great deal of thought and preparation needs to take place if such dietary restrictions are to be applied long-term.

When planning to, or undertaking a meat free/dairy free diet, it's best to get advice from qualified dieticians or those who have lived a vegetarian lifestyle for a long period.

It can also be a good idea to consult one of the many orthodox vegetarian societies too (preferably before beginning such a diet). They often have departments set up especially to assist persons who are new to, or contemplating a vegetarian lifestyle. With the help of such people, many of the risks associated with a vegetarian lifestyle can be reduced. Sadly however, all too often those who decide upon a vegetarian lifestyle have been influenced by newspaper/magazine articles and undertake such diets without any proper guidance at all.

SLIMMING AND EXERCISE

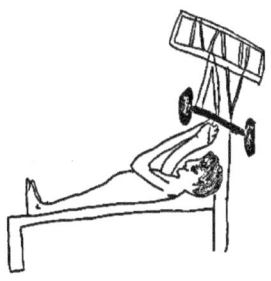

In recent times slimming and personal profile in terms of shape have very much been brought to our attention by way of the media and clothing designers. Our shape and appearance have become big business, but that does not necessarily make it right that our shape should rule the way we live. Despite all the hype about being slim and being healthy, recent evidence shows that there is only a small degree of truth in such claims, just as can apply to being slightly on the large size.

In a good many cases, our weight and shape have very little to do with our overall health **(provided we eat sensibly, in respect to portion size and types of meal, i.e. not too many burgers, pizzas, curries, pies**

and chips etc; or embark upon an extreme diet, whereby we become seriously underweight and malnourished).

Some people are meant to weigh 16 st/100kg; some people are meant to weigh 10 or 12st 60/80kg, 8st/50kg. We are all different; our metabolic rates vary tremendously, as do our frames and bodily structures.

We are only really have a problem if the following apply, i.e –

1. Where we have a consistently poor diet.

2. Where we have too much loose body fat hanging from our limbs/torso, or where we have been told by our medical practitioner or consultant to lose some weight on medical grounds, following cardio vascular tests etc.

3. Where our build and shape affect our self image and mental wellbeing.

It's true to a certain extent that we are what we eat, but not in all cases. Some people eat huge amounts of fatty food and put on hardly an ounce, whereas others need only small amounts of such foods to upset their tissue balance.

It's also true we all lay down body fat at different rates, but regardless of this, if we eat large amounts of saturated fats and they are not burned up through exercise, or we are lucky enough to be able to naturally expel any excess by way of an ultra efficient metabolism, more often than not any excess fat will be stored somewhere in the body.

Although they might not be visibly evident to us, such fatty deposits can often cause us serious internal health problems (by lining and clogging the arteries etc), so in all cases, it's best to keep our intake of high fat foods to a minimum, sticking instead to low fat dairy produce, white meat, fish etc wherever possible.

Despite the fact that we are now more aware of our need to restrict and control our diets and the fact that our saturated fat intake has tailed off considerably (in many cases either through our adopting a vegetarian or healthy eating regime); illnesses such as heart attacks have increased horrendously in recent years. This is mainly because we are not using our bodies enough.

Nowadays many of those calories which we do consume are being laid down as fat tissue in many cases. No matter whether they originate from dairy produce or carbohydrates, the outcome is often the same. Once we acknowledge this fact, loosing weight becomes much easier. It's no good to simply stop eating however. It's also important to undertake a suitable exercise programme as well, together with a suitable diet, as per the examples in the general health diet section of this document.

Some people advocate specialised diets consisting solely of fruit, vegetable, or a dairy-free diet. It's true such diets may help us to lose a degree of weight, but in denying ourselves a full range of foodstuffs, we risk a nutritional deficiency of some kind, or possibly an overdose of one type of nutrient. Eating too many bananas, could result in potassium poisoning for example; overdosing on carrot juice, cabbage juice etc can be just as dangerous). Even drinking too much water can be very dangerous in that it can thin our blood to a dangerous degree. None of these outcomes are desirable.

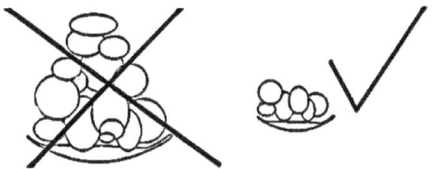

When seeking to lose weight (for whatever reason), it's best to simply reduce the amount of food we eat by having smaller portions of each foodstuff. This may sound like a very difficult thing to do, but it needn't be so if we load our plate strategically with salad materials (minus salad dressings).

It can also be a good idea to use a smaller plate for our meal too. As well as making our meal look more appetising, such a strategy also gives the impression that the plate is fuller. The best thing about salad based meals however is that we can eat fairly large quantities of them without putting on weight, besides that they are full of nutrients.

This tactic is not to everyone's taste of course, and so others will need to employ one of the other techniques available, such as attending regular exercise classes, or joining a local weight management group. Both of these options can be very effective, in that we have the support of those around us and can on occasion learn from their experiences.

Losing weight is generally a long-term operation, and so it's important to have support whilst we are trying to do so. It can often take a very long time before any real evidence of our efforts show through however.

Sadly it's only too easy to get disheartened when viewing the results attained by others, particularly those who have undertaken a quick fix diet of some kind, having adhered to a very harsh or selective diet. People who do lose weight in this way, often do so far too quickly and are inclined to suffer some degree of illness, as a result of starving themselves of essential nutrients.

It is also the case that those who undertake a quick fix or faddy diet often lose vast amounts of fluid, only to put weight back on again once they resume their normal diet. Others trying such methods are inclined to restrict their diet to such a degree that their craving for normal foodstuffs overwhelms them; starvation/restrictive diets are therefore not advisable.

Some people find keeping a diary in respect to their food intake and weight fluctuation helpful, in that they can see for themselves the effects of their efforts, and the way some foods affect them.

In all cases, establishing an exercise routine of some kind (suitable to our circumstances) will be crucial to our success. By far the most effective of these involve walking briskly, participating in some form of sport or swimming.

It is not good to exercise too vigorously in the early stages of our chosen exercise routine however, for its very likely our muscles ligaments and tendons will have become very weak through lack of use in the past. They could easily be damaged if we are too enthusiastic in our endeavours. It is therefore important to build up muscle tone over a period of weeks. It's often a good idea to enrol with an established exercise class where there is a qualified instructor present to direct and advise us, in respect to our routine.

By far the easiest and most pleasant form of exercise is of course massage by a professional therapist, many of whom carry out slimming treatments in a series of six or eight weekly sessions. There are many advantages to this form of treatment. Instead of working up a sweat and risking self-injury, we can lie back and relax, at least in the short term, whilst the treatment programme is in progress. The massage will be very effective in toning our muscles and mobilising our fat reserves so that they can be eliminated by the relevant organs.

Massage in itself is not a complete slimming treatment however. A degree of physical exercise on our part will still need to be undertaken when our treatment sessions come to an end, and of course we will still have to watch our diet. Massage is certainly the quickest way of getting noticeable improvements in our tissue structure, but such treatments can be very expensive.

Probably the best and most cost effective methods of losing weight are, as I referred to earlier, by reducing the size of the meals we consume and walking to the shops instead of using the car, or else take regular walks in the countryside. (In both cases, the walks will need to be fairly brisk if they are to be effective.) Cycling to work can be another option for some, though the road traffic can be rather hazardous and the weather is not always suitable.

Provided exercise is taken regularly (say 1½ hours per week, taken in ½ hour sessions, spread out during the week). Where most of us are concerned, it should not be too difficult to reach, and maintain a reasonable weight, without having to resort to more drastic dietary measures.

With the advent of the motor car, the computer and other such labour-saving devices, physical labour is becoming no more than a pastime (as in gardening for example). Sport and exercise are becoming something we have to do, not to support ourselves, but simply to repair the damage our modern diets and sedentary lifestyles are doing to us.

Heart attacks seem to be occurring more and more in the middle-aged members of our community. This is particularly so with businessmen and women, where an excess of stress and poor diet, complete with lack of exercise, often lead to serious metabolic dysfunction. How many of us now walk or cycle anywhere? We are all becoming too inactive for our own good. Our bodies were designed to move and be used. Fortunately some of us are now taking this into account when planning our daily routine, and are using sports centres and health clubs to keep fit, with more physical activity being undertaken.

We are now starting to cycle more both to our places to work and in a leisure context. This can only be a good thing in health terms (provided we are aware of; and mindful of other road users). The ironic thing is that in all too many cases, we are now having to pay to exercise our bodies - something our forefathers would never have believed. Fortunately we are also becoming wise to fast food and our diets appear to be improving. The days of junk food are numbered for those of us willing to acknowledge the principles of nutrition and rules of life.

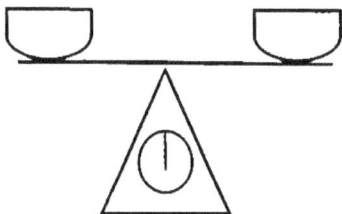

    The greatest rule in life, whether we are a judge or a tightrope walker or a man in the street, is balance; so it is with nutrition. Balance is the key to life. A balanced diet is the key to nutrition and good health.

CLOSING STATEMENT

Whilst it is hoped that the information in this guide has proved helpful, it is important to note however, that although a particular food or diet may be highly recommended by one particular body of experts at one point, it may be the case that another body of experts carrying out research, draw completely different conclusions in respect to a particular food's efficacy in respect to staving off certain types of illness; with the reverse being true in some cases. This has happened in respect to health scares regarding dairy produce, i.e. full cream milk, butter verses margarine, eggs, nutritional supplements etcetera. The same applies to wine and plain chocolate. Some see such products as detrimental to health, whilst others suggest they may be beneficial if consumed in moderation.

As with all advice and guidance; it cannot be stressed strongly enough that it is important to have good background knowledge in respect to any diet plans before undertaking them, which can involve a lot of research to find both the most effective and the safest option which is right for you. It is therefore up to all readers of this guide to seek out further in-depth information and use the most up to date research (via the internet etc) when seriously considering one of the dietary examples in this book or before commencing any of the specialised dietary examples in this book.

Acknowledgements

I would very much like to thank John R.S Allen for patiently helping me with the layout of this book and the many others who have helped me along the way.

www.ingramcontent.com/pod-product-compliance
Lightning Source LLC
Chambersburg PA
CBHW071550220526
45469CB00003B/967